Published By Adam Gilbin

@ Javier Ziebarth

Fodmap Diet: A Complete Guide to Create a Diet
Plan to Weight Loss and Wellness

All Right RESERVED

ISBN 978-1-990666-63-6

I0105873

TABLE OF CONTENTS

Blue Cheese And Arugula Salad With Red Wine Dressing

Ingredients:

- ½ English cucumber, sliced

- 1 avocado, pitted, peeled, and sliced (optional)

- ½ green bell pepper, seeded and thinly sliced

- 4 handfuls of arugula

- 1 cup (50 g) snow pea shoots or bean sprouts

- 7 ounces (200 g) blue cheese, cut into small chunks

Red wine dressing

- 2 tablespoons plus 2 teaspoons fresh lemon juice

- 1 tablespoon red wine vinegar

- 1 teaspoon gluten-free whole grain mustard

- 1 teaspoon sugar

- ¼ cup (60 ml) olive oil

- 2 heaping tablespoons chopped tarragon or flat-leaf parsley

Directions:

1. Combine the arugula, snow pea shoots, blue cheese, cucumber, avocado (if using), and bell pepper in a large bowl.
2. To make the dressing, combine all the ingredients in a small screw-top jar and shake until well mixed.
3. Just before serving, pour the dressing over the salad and gently toss to combine.

Smoked Chicken And Walnut Salad

Ingredients:

- 4 large hard-boiled eggs, halved

- 1 avocado, pitted, peeled, and sliced (optional)

- 14 ounces (400 g) smoked chicken or plain roast chicken, thinly sliced

- ¼ cup (25 g) toasted walnuts

- Salt and freshly ground black pepper

- ½ cup (150 g) gluten-free mayonnaise

- ½ teaspoon gluten-free soy sauce

- 3 tablespoons fresh lemon juice

- 2 heads baby romaine lettuce, leaves separated

- ½ cup (20 g) alfalfa sprouts

Directions:

1. To make the dressing, whisk together the mayonnaise, soy sauce, and lemon juice in a small bowl.
2. Combine the lettuce, sprouts, eggs, and avocado (if using) in a large salad bowl.
3. Drizzle the dressing over the top and toss gently to coat. Just before serving, add the chicken and walnuts, season to taste, and serve.

Vermicelli Salad With Chicken, Cilantro, And Mint

Ingredients:

- 10½ ounces (300 g) gluten-free rice vermicelli

Dressing

- 2 tablespoons light brown sugar

- ½ red chile pepper, seeded and finely chopped

- 1 tablespoon sesame oil

- 4⅓ cups (350 g) shredded cooked chicken breasts

- 2 tablespoons fresh lime juice

- 1 tablespoon fish sauce, or 2 teaspoons soy sauce and 1 extra teaspoon fresh lime juice

- Small handful of cilantro leaves, roughly chopped

- Small handful of mint leaves, roughly chopped

- Salt and freshly ground black pepper

Directions:

1. Fill a large bowl with very hot water.
2. Add the vermicelli and soak for 4 to 5 minutes, until softened.
3. Drain and rinse under cold water, then drain again.
4. To make the dressing, combine all the ingredients in a small screw-top jar and shake until well mixed.
5. Combine the noodles, chicken, cilantro, and mint in a large bowl.
6. Add the dressing, season to taste with salt and pepper, and toss well to combine.
7. Refrigerate for 2 to 3 hours before serving to allow the flavors to meld.

Low Fodmap Minestrone

Ingredients:

- 65g middle bacon & 80g (1 cup) leek

- 240g (2 large) carrot & 160g (1 small) potato

- 50g celery & 1 tbsp garlic infused oil

Drizzle of olive oil

- 400g plain crushed/chopped tomatoes

- 50 ml (2 cups) low FODMAP chicken stock/vegetable stock

- 310ml (1 1/4 cup) boiling water

- 12g (1/2 cup) fresh basil && 75g (1/2 cup) gluten free pasta 60g (2 cups) spinach & 160g zucchini

- 168 g (1 cup) canned chickpeas in brine

Directions:

1. Shakers the potato and carrot, finely reduce the celery, finely lower the inexperienced leek recommendations, and evacuate the pores and skin and cut the bacon into little pieces.

2. Spot a massive pan over medium warm temperature. Include the garlic injected oil, carrot, bacon, potato, celery, and green leek hints.

3. Saute tenderly for 15 to twenty minutes till the fixings begin to loosen up. Include a bath of olive oil and flip down the warm temperature if necessary.

4. While the veggies relax, dice the zucchinis, and daintily reduce the spinach leaves.

5. Make the low FODMAP stock if important. Channel and wash the chickpeas, before depleting yet again.

6. At that factor consist of the canned tomatoes, low FODMAP stock, high temp water, diced

zucchinis, spinach leaves, and chickpeas. Bring to the bubble and permit to stew on medium-low warmness for 10 mins.

7. Measure out the pasta and typically slash the basil (leaves and stalks). Save any little basil leaves for trimming.

8. Pour the pasta and basil to the soup.

9. Cook the pasta with the soup as indicated by means of parcel bearings, or until the pasta is done. if the soup is merely thick, keep adding water to your satisfaction.

10. Season with salt and pepper. Trimming with infant basil leaves and consist of a shower of garlic combined oil and a sprinkle of parmesan cheddar.

Low Fodmap Summer Beef Salad With Mustard Vinaigrette

Ingredients:

- 1 red bell peppers (deseeded & cut into strips) && 16 cherry tomato

- 10g (1/4 cup) green onions/scallions & Mustard Vinaigrette

- 1 ½ tbsp dijon mustard & 2 tbsp white vinegar

- 60ml (1/4 cup) olive oil & ¼ tsp black pepper

- ¼ tsp white sugar

- 1 tbsp neutral oil (rice bran, canola, sunflower)

- 600g beef rump steak & Season with salt & pepper

- 180g green beans & 6 cups lettuce (butter, iceberg, red coral)

Directions:

1. Cut the red ringer peppers into strips and flame broil in the broiler at 220ºC (440ºF) until the skins begin to darken.
2. Expel from broiler and permit to cool before stripping the external rankled skin off (this is the part that has gone dark).
3. While the red chime peppers cook you can do stages 2, 3 and 4.
4. Set up the green beans by evacuating the finishes and cutting into scaled down pieces. Wash and shred the lettuce before separating between the plates.
5. Split the cherry tomatoes and finely cut the green onions/scallions (green tips as it were). Put a little pot of water on to bubble.

6. Season the backside steak by scouring each side in the nonpartisan oil and salt and pepper.

7. Warmth a huge frypan over medium-high warmth and cook the steak for 3-4 minutes for each side for medium uncommon, or until cooked just as you would prefer.

8. Permit to rest for five minutes before daintily cutting.

9. While the steak cooks, you can whiten the green beans in bubbling water for two minutes (they ought to go brilliant green and delicate).

10. Channel and wash under virus water, at that point channel once more.

11. To make the mustard vinaigrette blend the dijon mustard, white vinegar, olive oil, sugar and dark pepper together until smooth.

12. On the off chance that the vinaigrette is too
    harsh take a stab at including two or three
    portions of sugar until it is sweet enough.
13. Amass the plate of mixed greens and serve
    the cut posterior steak on top, before
    showering in a mustard vinaigrette.

Healthy Fish & Chips With Tartare Sauce

Ingredients:

- Grated zest and juice 1 lemon

- Small handful of parsley leaves, chopped

- 1 tbsp capers , chopped

- 2 heaped tbsp 0% greek yogurt

- Lemon wedge, to serve

- 450g potatoes , peeled and cut into chips

- 1 tbsp olive oil , plus a little extra for brushing

- 2 white fish fillets about 140g/5oz each

Directions:

1. Heat oven to 200C/fan 180C/gas 6. Toss chips in oil.

2. Spread over a baking sheet in an even layer, bake for 40 mins until browned and crisp.

3. Put the fish in a shallow dish, brush lightly with oil, salt and pepper.

4. Sprinkle with half the lemon juice, bake for 12-15 mins.

5. After 10 mins sprinkle over a little parsley and lemon zest to finish cooking.

6. Meanwhile, mix the capers, yogurt, remaining parsley and lemon juice together, set aside and season if you wish.

7. To serve, divide the chips between plates, lift the fish onto the plates and serve with a spoonful of yogurt mix.

Perfect Scrambled Eggs Recipe

Ingredients:

- 2 large free range eggs

- 6 tbsp single cream or full cream milk

- A knob of butter

Directions:

1. Lightly whisk 2 large eggs, 6 tbsp single cream or full cream milk and a pinch of salt together until the mixture has just one consistency.

2. Heat a small non-stick frying pan for a minute or so, then add a knob of butter and let it melt.

3. Don't allow the butter to brown or it will discolour the eggs.

4. Pour in the egg mixture and let it sit, without stirring, for 20 seconds.

5. Stir with a wooden spoon, lifting and folding it over from the bottom of the pan.

6. Let it sit for another 10 seconds then stir and fold again.

7. Repeat until the eggs are softly set and slightly runny in places. Remove from the heat and leave for a moment to finish cooking.

8. Give a final stir and serve the velvety scramble without delay.

Thai-Style Rice And Meat Noodles

Ingredients:

- 200g sirloin steak

- 60g rice noodles

- 115g broccoli

- ½ carrot, grated

- 45g soybeans

- 1 tbsp mint, finely chopped

- Salt

- 1.5 tablespoons of lime juice

- 1 tbsp fish sauce

- 1 tbsp olive oil

- 1 tbsp sugar

- ½ chili

Directions:

1. Pour the lime juice, fish sauce, oil, sugar, and chili into a bowl.
2. Mix everything well.
3. Take 2 tablespoons of this marinade and put them in a bowl and set the rest aside.
4. Arrange the meat and turn it over to sprinkle it well with the marinade.
5. Cover and leave to rest in the refrigerator for an hour.
6. Cook the spaghetti and broccoli
7. Cook the spaghetti al dente in a pot of boiling salted water. Drain them and pour them into a bowl.
8. Cook the broccoli al dente in a pot of boiling salted water. Drain them and put them in the salad bowl.
9. Add the carrot, bean sprouts, and mint, season with the reserved marinade, and mix.

10. Cook the meat on the barbecue or in a pan and cut it into thin slices.

11. hen arrange them in the salad bowl.

Curried Carrot Soup

Ingredients:

- 1 tsp ground coriander

- 1/4 tsp dried chilli flakes (optional)

- 1/4 tsp ground ginger

- 1/2 tsp ground turmeric

- 1/4 tsp dried thyme

- 450g carrots (peeled and cut into small pieces)

- 1 potato (peeled and diced)

- 1.2 litres of vegetable stock (suitably low FODMAP)

- Salt and pepper to taste

For the croutons:

- 1/4 tsp ground pepper

- 2 tbsps vegetable oil

- 6 slices of gluten-free bread

- 1/4 tsp salt

Directions:

1. Prepare your vegetables as directed.

2. Place a large stock pot over a medium-high heat and put all of your Ingredients:into it. Leave it to simmer until the vegetables are tender.

3. While the soup is simmering make the croutons by cutting the bread into small cubes and placing them in a hot frying pan.

4. Drizzle the oil over the top of the bread and season with the salt and pepper before continually moving the croutons around the pan to ensure they toast evenly.

5. Once they're crispy remove them from the oven and keep them warm in a low temperature oven.

6. Using caution because the soup will be very hot, in small batches ladle some of the soup into your food processor or NutriBullet and blend until smooth. (Exercise caution when unscrewing the top of your NutriBullet because pressure will have built up inside due to the heat of the soup, so covering it with a tea towel before opening it would be highly advised.)

7. Once you've blended all of the soup serve it with the croutons.

A Hearty Corned Beef Soup

Ingredients:

- 3 potatoes

- 2 or 3 vegetable stock cubes (to taste) (suitably low FODMAP)

- 1.5 litres of hot water

- 2 tins of good quality corned beef

- 3 large carrots

Directions:

1. Chop up your vegetables into bite-sized pieces (or grate them) and put them in a large soup pot.
2. Add enough hot water so it just covers the vegetables and bring to the boil.
3. Chop up your corned beef and add it to the pot.

4. Simmer gently until your veg is cooked and then add the stock cubes one at a time, tasting after stirring each one in to make sure you don't over-season the soup. (You might not need all 3 stock cubes, depending on your personal taste.)
5. After simmering it for a wee while longer serve it with good gluten-free bread and butter.

Individual Strawberry & Rhubarb Quinoa Crumbles

Ingredients:

- 140g gluten-free oats

- 45g quinoa flakes

- 65g walnuts, chopped

- 2 tsp cinnamon

- 3 tbsp coconut oil, melted

- 1 tsp pure vanilla extract

- 200g rhubarb

- 400g strawberries, hulled

- Juice of ½ a lime

- 6 tbsp maple syrup

- 1 tbsp brown sugar to top (optional)

- Lactose-free cream to serve (optional)

Directions:

1. Preheat the oven to 180°C (gas 4). Grease individual tins or ramekins with a little coconut oil and put to one side.

2. Chop the rhubarb, slice the strawberries, and place in a large bowl.

3. Add the lime juice and 2 tablespoons of the maple syrup and stir to combine.

4. Divide the fruit among the ramekins.

5. To make the crumble, put the oats, quinoa flakes, walnuts and cinnamon in a large bowl and stir to combine.

6. Add the coconut oil, remaining 4 tablespoons of maple syrup and vanilla extract and stir once more.

7. Spoon the crumble mixture on top of the fruit in each dish and sprinkle with a little brown sugar if desired.

8. Bake for 2530 minutes, or until the crumble is golden brown and the fruit is bubbling.

9. Serve warm with a generous dollop of lactose-free cream.

Rich Chocolate Tart With A Chia Seed Base

Ingredients:

For the tart case

- ½ tsp sea salt

- 1 egg

- 30g lactose-free butter, melted

- 150g gluten-free flour blend

- 100g buckwheat flour

- 40g chia seeds

- A little extra butter or coconut oil, for greasing

For the filling

- 1 tbsp tapioca flour

- 250g dark (70%) chocolate

- 1 tsp pure vanilla extract

- 150ml almond milk

- 200ml water

- 75g brown sugar

Directions:

1. Preheat the oven to 180°C (gas 4) and lightly grease a 20cm round tart tin.
2. In a mixing bowl, combine the flours, chia seeds and sea salt. Stir to combine.
3. Whisk the egg and add to the dry ingredients along with the melted butter. Stir with a wooden spoon, then using your hands, knead the dough until it comes together.
4. Push the dough into the tart tin base until roughly 5mm thick.
5. Prick the base all over with a fork and place in the oven. Bake for 15 minutes, or until lightly

golden. Remove from the oven and allow to cool slightly.

6. To make the filling, place the milk in a small saucepan with the water and sugar.

7. Warm over a low heat. Put the tapioca flour in a small bowl with a few tablespoons of the warm milk mixture and stir until smooth.

8. Add the mixture to the pan, stir and bring to the boil, before taking off the heat.

9. Break the chocolate into a bowl and pour over the hot milk mixture; stir until smooth and creamy.

10. Add the vanilla extract and a pinch of sea salt, then pour into the tart case and chill for 56 hours before serving.

Mango Salsa

Ingredients:

- 2 tablespoons chopped fresh lime juice

- 1 teaspoon salt

- 1/2 teaspoon black pepper

- 1 mango

- 1 red onion

- 1 jalapeño pepper

- 2 tablespoons chopped cilantro

Directions:

1. Cut the mango into small cubes.
2. Peel and chop the red onion.
3. Slice the jalapeño pepper into thin strips.

4. In a medium bowl, combine the mango, red onion, jalapeño pepper, cilantro, lime juice, salt and black pepper.

5. Serve immediately or store in a covered container in the fridge for later use.

Celery Root Tahini Dip

Ingredients:

- 1/2 small red onion, diced

- 1 tbsp. Extra virgin olive oil

- 1 garlic clove, minced

- 1 cup tahini

- 1 celery root, peeled and diced

- Salt and pepper to taste

Directions:

1. In a medium bowl, whisk together the tahini, celery root, red onion, olive oil and garlic.
2. Season with salt and pepper to taste.
3. Serve with chips or crackers.

Basic Nut Or Seed Pâté

Ingredients:

- 1 tablespoon of oil

- 1 teaspoon of salt

- 1 cup of nuts or seeds

Directions:

1. Preheat the oven to 350 degrees Fahrenheit.
2. Spread the nuts or seeds onto a baking sheet and bake for 10-15 minutes, until lightly toasted.
3. In a small skillet, heat the oil over medium heat.
4. Add the salt and stir until the salt is fully dissolved.
5. Pour the salted oil onto the toasted nuts or seeds and toss to coat. Serve immediately!

Garlic-Infused Oil

Ingredients:

- 8 garlic cloves peeled and crushed

- 1 teaspoon red pepper flakes (optional)

- 1 cup olive oil

Directions:

1. Heat the oil in a heavy-gauge pot over medium heat.
2. Add the garlic and red pepper flakes (if using). Cook until aromatic, 2 to 3 minutes.
3. Remove from the heat. Let cool to room temperature.
4. Strain the oil into a clean jar. Discard the garlic and red pepper flakes.
5. Store the oil in the refrigerator for up to 7 days.

Tostadas

Ingredients:

- 1 cup diced tomatoes (canned or fresh)

- Salt and freshly ground black pepper

- 8 tostada shells (gluten-free)

- 1 cup grated aged sharp Cheddar cheese

- 2 green onions (green part only), minced

- 1 tablespoon olive oil

- 1 pound lean ground turkey

- 2 teaspoons chili powder (garlic-free)

- 1 teaspoon ground cumin

Directions:

1. Preheat the oven to 325°F. Heat the oil in a large cast-iron skillet over high heat.

2. Add the ground turkey. Sauté, stirring frequently, until the meat is evenly cooked and browned, 6 to 8 minutes.

3. Add the chili powder and cumin, and stir to combine.

4. Add the tomatoes. Cook, stirring occasionally, until thickened and flavorful, 10 to 12 minutes. Season with salt and pepper.

5. Place the tostada shells on two baking sheets.

6. Divide the turkey mixture, cheese, and green onions evenly among the shells.

7. Bake until the cheese is melted and bubbly, 8 to 10 minutes.

Pineapple-Coconut Smoothie

Ingredients:

- 1 cup unsweetened almond milk

- 1 cup crushed ice

- 2 tablespoons chia seeds or flaxseed

- 2 cups crushed pineapple, fresh or canned in water and drained

- 1 cup canned full-fat coconut milk

Directions:

1. In a blender, combine the pineapple, coconut milk, almond milk, ice, and chia seeds.
2. Blend until smooth.

Strawberry Smoothie

Ingredients:

- ½ cup FODMAP-approved milk (almond milk is recommended)

- ⅔ cup strawberries, fresh or frozen

- ¼ cup lactose-free yogurt or vegan yogurt

- 1 ½ tsp protein powder

- 1 tsp chia seeds

- ½ tbsp maple syrup

- 1 tsp lemon juice

- ¼ tsp vanilla extract

- 6 ice cubes (only when using fresh strawberries)

Directions:

1. Cut the strawberries into halves or quarters. If using frozen strawberries, it is recommended to cut them the day before.

2. Put Ingredients:into a blender and blend until smooth. If the mixture gets too thick, add a small amount of hot water and continue blending.

3. It is best drunk immediately.

Dilly Egg Salad

Ingredients:

- ½ teaspoon dill, dried

- 1 tablespoon mayonnaise

- Salt and pepper

- 4 hard-boiled eggs, peeled and chopped

- 1 tablespoon spicy mustard

Directions:

1. Place all of the Ingredients:in a bowl. Mix well.
2. Season to taste.

Pumpkin Pancakes

Ingredients:

- ½ teaspoon vanilla

- 1 large egg

- ¼ teaspoon baking powder

- 2 tablespoons coconut flour

- ½ firm banana, mashed

- ½ teaspoon pumpkin pie spice

- ¼ cup pumpkin puree

Directions:

1. Combine pumpkin and banana together in a bowl. Mix well.
2. Add remaining Ingredients:. Stir well until smooth.

3. Pour mixture in a pan. Cook over medium heat in oil for 5 minutes on each side. Repeat procedure for the remaining mixture.

Eggplant Stuffed With Tomato With Tzatziki

Ingredients:

- 1 piece of finely chopped onion

- 3 garlic cloves finely chopped

- 1 tablespoon cinnamon powder

- 1 tablespoon ground cumin

- 1 tablespoon of tomato puree

- 4 pieces of tomato cut into medium cubes

- 1 tablespoon of agave honey

- 1 pinch of salt

- 1 pinch of pepper

- 1/4 cup of lemon juice

- 1 bunch of finely chopped parsley

- 1/2 bunch of finely chopped parsley

- 4 Portions

- 2 pieces of medium aubergine, cut in half, frayed

- 3 tablespoons olive oil

- 1/2 cup of soy yogurt

- 1 clove garlic

- 3 tablespoons finely chopped mint

- 1 pinch of paprika

Directions:

1. Preheat the oven to 200 ° C
2. Heat a small pot at medium heat with the oil, sauté the onion with the garlic, add the ground cinnamon, the cumin, the tomato puree, the tomato, and the agave honey, cook for 10 minutes, season to your liking.

3. In a table, aubergines are filled and stuffed with the tomato sautéed, baked in a tray for 20 minutes.
4. Remove from the oven and reserve.
5. To form the tzatziki in a bowl mix the lemon juice, with the parsley, the cucumber, the yogurt, the garlic, the mint, and the paprika.
6. Mix until a homogeneous mixture is formed.
7. Serve the aubergines with the Turkish sauce and serve with a bit of pita bread or unleavened bread.

Eggplant Chips

Ingredients:

- 1/4 cup of coconut milk

- 1/3 cup of onion chambray only the tail and cut into rings, for the dip

- 1 tablespoon chopped chipotle chili, for the dip

- 1/4 cup of toasted pinion, for the dip

- 1 pinch of salt for the dip

- 10 Portions

- 2 pieces of eggplant cut into thin strips, torn, washed and dried

- 1/4 cup of goat cheese for a dip

- 1/4 cup of cream cheese

- 1 pinch of pepper for the dip

Directions:

1. Preheat oven to 160 ° C
2. In a tray spread the eggplant slices and bake for 20 minutes, remove from the oven turn the aubergines and bake for 20 minutes or until they are dehydrated and crispy.
3. Remove it from the oven and then let it cool the chips.
4. In a bowl mix the creamy goat cheese with cream cheese and coconut milk, add the onion Cambray, the chipotle chili minced, the pine nuts and season to taste with salt and pepper.
5. Combine the aubergines with the dip and enjoy.

Fody's Korean Bbq Shrimp Lettuce Wraps

Ingredients:

- 1 Tbsp

- Fody Shallot-Infused Olive Oil

- 2 Tbsp

- 1/2 cup brown rice, dry

- 18-24 shrimp, thawed, deveined + tails removed

- 1/2 cup carrots, shredded (~2 carrots)

- 1/4 cup celery, diced

- 1/4 cup green onion tops, diced

- Fody Korean BBQ Sauce

- Salt + pepper, to taste

- 6 leaves of lettuce (use Bibb, Butter, Romaine, etc. anything that makes a good cup)

- Optional garnish: chopped peanuts, sesame seeds

Directions:

1. Cook rice according to package Directions: (TIP: prep veggies while rice cooks!)
2. Pat shrimp dry and add to small bowl. Toss in Fody Shallot-Infused or Garlic-Infused Olive Oil, salt, and pepper.
3. Heat pan over medium-high and cook shrimp, 1-2 mins per side until pink.
4. Remove shrimp from heat and add to a clean bowl. Toss in Fody Korean BBQ Sauce.
5. When rice is cooked, stir in shredded carrots, diced celery, and green onion until well-combined. Season with salt and pepper.
6. Plate lettuce wraps and top with rice mixture.

7. Add shrimp, 3-4 pieces per cup. Garnish with chopped peanuts and sesame seeds.
8. Serve with extra Korean BBQ Sauce for dipping. Enjoy your Low FODMAP lettuce wraps!

Fody's Gluten-Free Baked Funfetti Donuts

Ingredients:

- 4 tbsp almond oil (or other neutral oil)

- 4 tbsp almond milk

- 2 tsp vanilla

- ½ tsp almond extract

- ¼ tsp nutmeg

- ¼ tsp salt

- 4 large eggs

- ¼ cup sprinkles (Low FODMAP sprinkles)

- ⅔ cup powdered sugar

- ¾ cup coconut cream

- 1 tsp vanilla

- Extra sprinkles for garnish (Low FODMAP sprinkles)

- 2 cups almond flour

- ⅔ cup sugar

- 2 tsp baking powder

- ½ cup tapioca flour

Directions:

1. Pre-heat the oven to 350F and grease a silicone donut pan.
2. In a large mixing bowl add eggs, sugar, vanilla, almond extract, almond oil and milk + beat until smooth.
3. Next add almond flour, baking powder, tapioca flour, nutmeg, salt & sprinkles to the wet ingredients. Using a silicone spatula, fold

dry ingredients into wet until fully
incorporated.

4. If your batter has some clumps, gently whisk
    until no clumps remain, being careful not to
    over mix the batter.

5. Pour batter into a silicone donut pan and
    place the donut pan on a baking sheet for
    easier in and out of the oven.

6. Bake for 15 minutes or until a toothpick
    comes out clean.

7. While donuts bake, whisk together powdered
    sugar, coconut cream, and vanilla until a
    smooth glaze forms.

8. Allow donuts to cool completely prior to
    glazing. Once baked donuts are cool, dip them
    top down into the glaze. Sprinkle with
    additional Low FODMAP sprinkles if desired.

Vegetable Soup

Ingredients:

- 2 large carrots, cut into chunks

- 14 ounces (400 g) kabocha or other suitable winter squash, peeled, seeded, and cut into chunks

- 3 potatoes, cut into chunks

- 4 cups (1 liter) gluten-free, onion-free vegetable stock*

- 1½ cups (375 ml) low-fat milk, lactose-free milk, or suitable plant-based milk

- 2 tablespoons garlic-infused olive oil

- 2 celery stalks, tough strings removed, halved lengthwise and cut into ¼-inch (5 mm) slices

- 1 head broccoli, cut into chunks (including stalks)

- 3 rutabagas, peeled and cut into chunks

- Salt and freshly ground black pepper

Directions:

1. Heat the oil in a large heavy-bottomed stockpot over medium heat. Add the celery and cook, stirring, until golden brown. Add the broccoli, rutabagas, carrots, squash, and potatoes. Pour in the stock. Bring to a boil, reduce the heat, and simmer, covered, for 1 hour or until the vegetables are tender.

2. Remove from the heat and leave to cool to room temperature. Use an immersion blender to puree the vegetables to a smooth consistency. (Alternatively, carefully transfer the vegetables to a food processor and process until smooth.)

3. Stir in the milk, season to taste with salt and pepper, and reheat gently.

Spicy Clear Soup

Ingredients:

- 6½ cups (1.5 liters) gluten-free, onion-free chicken or vegetable stock

- 2 tablespoons plus 2 teaspoons fish sauce, or 4 teaspoons soy sauce and 2 teaspoons fresh lime juice

- 1 tablespoon plus 1 teaspoon fresh lime juice

- 3 bunches baby bok choy, quartered, rinsed, and drained

- 2 heaping tablespoons chopped cilantro

- One 8-ounce (225 g) can bamboo shoots, drained

- One 14-to 15-ounce (400 g) can baby corn, drained, or 7½ ounces (215 g) fresh baby corn, cut on the diagonal (about 1½ cups/360 ml)

- 3½ ounces (100 g) gluten-free rice vermicelli (about 2 cups)

- 1 tablespoon sesame oil

- 2 teaspoons garlic-infused olive oil

- 2 teaspoons rice bran oil or sunflower oil

- 2 heaping tablespoons finely chopped lemongrass (white portion only)

- ½ to 1 red chile pepper, seeded and finely chopped

- 6 pieces dried galangal root (optional)

Directions:

1. Heat the sesame oil, garlic-infused oil, and rice bran oil in a large saucepan over medium heat.

2. Add the lemongrass and chile and cook for 2 minutes or until fragrant.

3. Add the galangal (if using), stock, fish sauce, and lime juice and bring to a boil.

4. Add the bok choy, cilantro, bamboo shoots, baby corn, and vermicelli.

5. Reduce the heat and simmer for 3 minutes or until the vegetables and noodles are tender. (Remove the galangal.) Serve immediately.

Carrot & Corn Fritters

Ingredients:

- 240g (2 large) carrot & 1 red bell peppers (large)

- 12g (1/4 cup) fresh chives & 2 tbsp fresh parsley

- 128g (3/4 cup) sweet corn

- Carrot & Corn Fritters & 2 large egg

- 63ml (1/4 cup) low FODMAP milk

- 70g (1/2 cup) gluten free all purpose flour

- ½ tsp ground cumin & 1 ½ tsp paprika

Directions:

1. Mesh the carrots, deseed and dice the crimson ringer peppers, and degree out the

corn quantities. Nicely cleave the chives and parsley.

2. In a big bowl mix the eggs and espresso milk (FODMAP) together.

3. Whilst you are carried out with that mixture inside the flour, paprika, and cumin.

4. Mix the corn, carrot, pink ringer peppers, chives, and parsley until they form. Season with salt and pepper.

5. Spot a massive non-stick fry container over medium warm temperature and shower with oil.

6. Spoon 1/four cup combo for each waste into the container.

7. Cook 4 to six wastes one after some other leveling them marginally so they are not very thick.

8. Permit to cook dinner for 3 to 4mins for every aspect, till extremely good dark-colored and cooked through.

9. Ensure you blend the blend before cooking each bunch.

10. Serve 3 wastes for everybody.

Pork Loin Roast With Herb Stuffing

Ingredients:

- 1 tbsp garlic infused oil & 1 cup fresh parsley

- 10g (1/4 cup) green onions/scallions

- 1 tsp dried oregano & ½ tsp dried thyme

- 3 tbsp pumpkin seeds & Season with rock salt

- 2.5kg pork loin roast & 200g medium-grain white rice

- 500ml (2 cups) low FODMAP chicken stock

- 120g (1 1/2 cup) leek & 1 tbsp olive oil

Directions:

1. Make the risotto. Generally, curb the inexperienced leek recommendations. Make the bird inventory with effervescent water if utilizing stock three-D shapes. Warmth a big

pan over medium warmth. Fry the leek hints in the olive oil and garlic implanted the oil for 2 minutes. Include the Arborio rice, mix thru the mixture for around 1 moment.

2. Next, include 125mls (half cup) of hen inventory straight away, mix from time to time until the fluid has ingested into the rice. Continue which includes and mixing in the stock, a sprinkle without delay. Turn down the warm temperature to medium-low if essential. When the rice has fed on two cups of inventory, take a look at and take a look at whether the rice is cooked (need to take around 20 minutes). On the off threat that it is not, encompass more and more stock and maintain cooking for an additional few minutes. You want the rice to be cooked and sticky however not very wet. While the risotto chefs, finely hack the parsley and inexperienced onions/scallions.

3. Take the rice from the warm temperature and mix via the parsley, inexperienced onions/scallions, dried oregano, thyme, and pumpkin seeds. Move to a plastic holder or bowl and allow to chill.

4. Stuff and tie your pork cook. In the occasion that viable take the stuffing to the butcher and get them to stuff and tie the beef flank cook dinner for you. Request that they score the pores and skin and fats for you too.

5. In the occasion which you cannot do this watch those recordings. They will show you a way to stuff and tie the meal. Before you stuff the meal you do want to score the skin with a pointy blade about 1cm/½ inch down and approximately 1cm/½ inch separated. Discover the way to reduce a pork flank cook right here (watch until 2mins 30 seconds).

6. The best technique to tie up the red meat prepare dinner here.

7. Cook your pork. Preheat the range to 220ºC (430ºF) fan warmth paintings. Rub the pork pores and skin with olive oil and season liberally with salt. Spot in a broiling plate and circulate into the broiler as soon as hot. Broil for 30 minutes. Expel from broiler and deal with with the pork juices (sprinkle the pork squeezes over the meal) and daintily season once more with salt.

8. Turn down the stove warm temperature to 200ºC (390ºF) and broil the pork for about an extra 1 hour and 30 minutes. Season the pork like clockwork. On the off chance that your snapping is cooking excessively brief or seems as though it is able to devour then unfold it with tinfoil. Your dish may additionally take marginally longer to cook contingent upon the appropriate size. Expel the red meat from the broiler whilst the snapping is superb and the

juices run clean (embed a pointy blade into the meal).

9. Rest for 10mins earlier than slicing. Present with your selected facets of greens and natively built cranberry sauce.

Potato Salad With Anchovy & Quail's Eggs

Ingredients:

- 1 anchovy , finely chopped

- 1 tbsp chopped parsley

- 1 tbsp chopped chives

- juice 0.5 lemon

- 4 quail's eggs

- 100g green beans

- 100g new potatoes , halved or quartered if very large

Directions:

1. Bring a medium pan of water to a simmer. Lower the quail's eggs into the water and cook for 2 mins. Lift out the eggs with a slotted spoon and put into a bowl of cold

water. Add the beans to the pan, simmer for 4 mins until tender, then remove from the pan with a slotted spoon and plunge into the bowl of cold water.

2. Put the potatoes in the pan and boil for 10-15 mins until tender.

3. Drain the potatoes in a colander and leave them to cool.

4. While the potatoes are cooling, peel the eggs and cut them in half.

5. Toss the potatoes and beans with the chopped anchovy, herbs and lemon juice. Top with the quail's eggs to serve.

Gluten-Free Carrot Cake

Ingredients:

- 200g gluten-free self-raising flour

- 1 tsp cinnamon

- 1 tsp gluten-free baking powder

- 50g mixed nut , chopped

- 140g unsalted butter , softened, plus extra for greasing

- 200g caster sugar

- 250g carrots , grated

- 140g sultanas

- 2 eggs , lightly beaten

For the icing

- 75g butter , softened

- 175g icing sugar

- 3 tsp cinnamon , plus extra for dusting

Directions:

1. Heat oven to 180C/160C fan/gas 4. Grease and line a 900g/2lb loaf tin with baking parchment

2. Beat the butter and sugar until soft and creamy, then stir in the grated carrot and sultanas. Pour the eggs into the mix a little at a time.

3. Add the flour, cinnamon, baking powder and most of the chopped nuts and mix well.

4. Tip the mix into the loaf tin, then bake for 50-55 mins or until a skewer poked in the middle comes out clean. Allow to cool in the tin for 15 mins, then remove from the tin and cool completely on a wire rack.

5. Meanwhile, make the icing.

6. Beat the butter in a large bowl until it is really soft, add the icing sugar and cinnamon, then beat until thick and creamy.

7. When the cake is cool, spread the icing on top, then sprinkle with a little more cinnamon and the remaining chopped nuts.

Chicken Caesar Salad

Ingredients:

- 1 teaspoon Tabasco sauce

- 1 tablespoon vinegar

- 20 g bacon, diced

- 1/2 romaine lettuce Salt

- Pepper

- 2 tablespoons grated Parmesan

- 300g of chicken breast

- 3 tablespoons of flavored oil garlic

- 2 chopped anchovy fillets

- 1 yolk

- 1 teaspoon mustard

Directions:

1. You can cook the chicken on the barbecue or on the grill of a preheated oven.
2. Sprinkle the chicken with a little oil, salt, and pepper and cook for about ten minutes, turning it halfway through cooking.
3. When it is well cooked and golden, place it on a cutting board and cover it with aluminum foil.
4. Pour a tablespoon of garlic-flavored oil into a saucepan over low heat.
5. Add the anchovies, stirring with a spoon for a minute until they are dissolved.
6. Put the egg yolks in a bowl, along with the mustard, Tabasco sauce, and vinegar. Stir vigorously with a fork and then slowly
7. pour in the garlic-flavored oil, whisking until emulsion.
8. Add the oil with the anchovies and season with salt and pepper.

9. Heat the bacon in a non-stick pan. Once browned, place it on absorbent paper to remove some fat.

10. Wash and dry the lettuce and put it in a salad bowl after having cut it up.

11. Incorporate the bacon, and season it with the sauce, and mix well.

12. Cut thin slices of chicken and place them on the salad. Sprinkle with Parmesan and serve.

Poached Eggs And Ham

Ingredients:

- ½ tablespoon olive oil

- ½ tablespoon white vinegar

- ½ orange

- 15 g butter

- 2 tablespoons white wine

- 1 tablespoon Cointreau, or Grand Marnier

- (optional)

- 130g smoked ham, cut into 4 slices

- ½ teaspoon of chives, chopped

- 200g of potatoes

- 3 eggs

- 6 cl of cream cooking

- 5g dill, chopped

- Salt

- Pepper

Directions:

1. Prepare the potato mash
2. Bring to a boil the potatoes whole, without peeling, until very tender (about 20 minutes).
3. Drain them, peel them while still hot, put them in a bowl, and mash them well.
4. In a bowl, beat 2 eggs and then add them to the potatoes. Add the cooking cream, dill, a pinch of salt, and pepper.
5. Mix well and then let it cool until it is compact enough to form two flatbreads.
6. Heat the oil over medium-high heat in a heavy-bottomed skillet. Then put the

flatbreads and cook for 3-4 minutes on the side, until golden brown.

7. Put them on a plate and keep them warm in the oven.

8. Prepare the poached eggs

9. Fill a shallow, large saucepan with water.Add the vinegar and bring to a gentle boil over low heat.

10. Drop one egg at a time into the water. The egg is ready after about 3 minutes when the egg white has completely congealed assuming its white color (the yolk must instead be soft inside). Keep the eggs warm on a plate in the oven.

11. Assemble the final dish the flatbreads lace On individual plates (possibly hot), and put a slice of ham on top and the egg on top.

Lentil And Vegetable Soup

Ingredients:

- 2-3 vegetable stock cubes (suitably low FODMAP)

- 1 litre of boiling water

- 1 bouquet garni sachet

- Salt and pepper (to taste)

- 180g of tinned lentils (drained and rinsed well)

- 500g parsnips (grated)

- 500g carrots (grated)

Directions:

1. Drain and rinse the tinned lentils (this process helps to reduce their FODMAP content) and add them to a large soup pan.

2. Dissolve the stock cubes in a litre of boiling water and add the stock to the large soup pan along with all of the other Ingredients:.

3. Simmer the soup until the vegetables are soft and then taste, season with salt and pepper and serve. (You can add more boiling water if you'd like a looser soup.)

Cardamom Rice Pudding

Ingredients:

- 1 litre lactoseor dairy-free milk of choice (I like rice for a natural sweetness)

- 20g lactose-free butter, plus extra for greasing

- Toasted coconut, to serve

- 150g pudding rice

- 10 cardamom pods, lightly crushed

- 50g brown sugar

Directions:

1. Preheat the oven to 150°C (gas 2) and lightly butter a 1.5 litre ovenproof dish.
2. Into the dish toss the rice, cardamom pods and sugar.

3. Stir in the milk, dot with the butter and put in the oven.
4. Cook the pudding for 30 minutes then give it a stir.
5. Return to the oven for a further 30 minutes before stirring again.
6. Return to the oven for a final hour; by this time the rice should be tender and creamy.
7. Serve hot with a handful of toasted nuts or coconut.

Melon Sorbet

Ingredients:

- 4 tbsp maple syrup

- 4 tbsp water

- Dried edible flowers, to decorate

- 700g honeydew melon (roughly 1 large melon), chopped and frozen

- 1 tbsp lime juice

Directions:

1. Add all of the ingredients into a food processor and whizz until smooth.
2. Spoon into bowls and decorate with dried edible flowers.
3. Keep any leftovers back in the freezer for subsequent munching.

Papaya, Macadamia & Lime Salad

Ingredients:

- 450g lactoseor dairy-free yoghurt

- The zest of 1 lime, plus 2 limes to serve

- 2 small papayas

- 50g macadamia nuts

Directions:

1. Cut the papayas in half lengthways and scoop out the seeds.
2. Lightly crush the macadamia nuts in a pestle and mortar.
3. Spoon yoghurt into the papaya hollows, and sprinkle over the nuts and lime zest.
4. Serve immediately with extra lime wedges.

Lemon Gone Wild Dressing

Ingredients:

- 1 teaspoon salt

- 1/4 teaspoon black pepper

- 1/4 cup chopped fresh parsley

- 1/4 cup chopped fresh basil

- 1/2 cup olive oil

- 1/2 cup lemon juice

- 1 tablespoon Dijon mustard

- 1 tablespoon honey

Directions:

1. In a medium bowl, whisk together the olive oil, lemon juice, Dijon mustard, honey, salt and black pepper.

2. Pour the dressing into a small container and stir in the parsley and basil.

Bacon And Zucchini Crustless Quiche

Ingredients:

- 1 tsp salt

- 1/4 tsp black pepper

- 1/4 cup shredded cheddar cheese

- 1/4 cup shredded mozzarella cheese

- 8 biscuits (or 2 cups of Bisquick)

- 1 zucchini

- 1/2 lb bacon, diced

- 1 egg

- 1/4 cup milk

Directions:

1. Preheat oven to 375 degrees F. Grease a 9 inch pie dish with cooking spray.
2. Cut the zucchini into 1 inch thick slices and then slice the bacon into thin strips.
3. In a medium bowl, whisk together the egg, milk, salt and pepper.
4. Pour the mixture into the pie dish and top with the cheddar cheese and mozzarella cheese.
5. Bake for 25 minutes or until golden brown.
6. Serve hot with biscuit halves as an appetizer or dessert.

Stuffed Endive

Ingredients:

- 8 leaves Belgian endive

- ½ cup minced fresh flat-leaf parsley or fresh chives

- Freshly ground black pepper

- 12 ounces Brie or Camembert cheese, rind removed

- 2 green onions (green part only), minced

Directions:

1. Blend the Brie and green onions in a medium bowl with a wooden spoon or in a food processor until evenly combined.
2. Fill the endive leaves with the Brie-onion mixture.

3. Sprinkle with parsley and season with pepper. Serve immediately.

Flatbreads For Pizza

Ingredients:

- ½ cup almond milk

- 2 teaspoons lemon juice

- 2 teaspoons minced rosemary (optional)

- ½ teaspoon freshly ground black pepper (optional)

- 2 teaspoons clarified butter or ghee

- 1½ cups oat flour, plus more for rolling

- ⅔ cups tapioca flour

- ¼ cups brown rice flour

- ½ teaspoon baking powder

- ½ teaspoon sea salt

Directions:

1. In a large bowl, combine the oat flour, tapioca flour, brown rice flour, baking powder, and salt.

2. In a small bowl, combine the almond milk and lemon juice, and let sit for a few minutes to curdle.

3. To the flour mixture, add the curdled milk, rosemary (if using), and pepper (if using) and stir to make a stiff dough.

4. Divide the dough into four equal pieces. Working with one piece of dough at a time, roll out into disks on a well-floured work surface with a rolling pin, about ½ inch thick and 7 or 8 inches in diameter.

5. Coat the dough and rolling pin with additional oat flour as needed to prevent sticking.

6. Heat the clarified butter in a large cast-iron skillet over medium-high heat. Add one flatbread to the skillet.

7. Cook on the first side until golden brown, 6 to 7 minutes. Turn and cook on the second side until golden brown and cooked through, 2 to 3 minutes.

8. Repeat with the remaining flatbreads.

9. Serve immediately. The flatbreads can be prepared in advance.

10. Store in an airtight container in the refrigerator for up to 3 days or in the freezer for up to 2 months.

Orange-Scented Overnight Oatmeal

Ingredients:

- ¼ teaspoon cinnamon

- ½ teaspoon vanilla extract

- ¼ teaspoon orange extract

- ⅛ teaspoon ground ginger

- 1 cup gluten-free rolled oats

- 1¼ cups lactose-free milk, divided

- Juice of ½ orange

- ½ tablespoon chia seeds

- 1 tablespoon maple syrup, divided

Directions:

1. In a medium bowl, stir together the oats, 1 cup of the milk, orange juice, chia seeds, half

of the maple syrup, cinnamon, vanilla and orange extracts, and ginger.

2. Cover and refrigerate overnight.

3. To serve, stir in the remaining maple syrup, and serve chilled or warmed.

Baked Roasted Garlic Cabbage

Ingredients:

- 5 large garlic cloves, chopped

- Sea salt with freshly ground black pepper to taste

- 1 large green cabbage, slice into 1 "thick slices

- 3 tablespoons of virgin olive oil (use can use melted ghee)

Directions:

1. Preheat the oven to 204 C.
2. Brush both sides of each slice of cabbage with olive oil or ghee.
3. Sprinkle the garlic evenly on each side of the cabbage slices and season them to taste with salt and pepper.

4. Roast inside the oven for 20 minutes, then flip the slices and roast again for another 20 minutes or till the edges are crispy.

Fody's Low Fodmap Sesame Ginger Chicken With Coconut Rice

Ingredients:

- 2 2 ½ lbs boneless skinless chicken thighs, cubed

- 2 tbsp

- Fody's Shallot-Infused Olive Oil

- ¼ cup tapioca starch

- ½ tsp ground ginger

- ⅓ cup

- Fody's Sesame Ginger Marinade

- ¼ cup coconut aminos

- 1 tbsp sesame seeds

- 1 ½ cups white rice, uncooked

- 1 tsp sugar

- 1 14oz can full fat coconut milk

- 1 cup water

- Pinch of sea salt

- 1 cup snow peas (about 20 pods)

- Chopped scallion greens for garnish

Directions:

1. Bring water for rice to a boil over medium-high heat. Once water is boiling, add in rice + cook according to package instructions.

2. While rice cooks, whisk together Fody Sesame Ginger Marinade, coconut aminos, and sesame seeds in a medium bowl. Set aside.

3. In a large mixing bowl, whisk together tapioca starch + ground ginger and set aside.

4. Cube chicken thighs into ½" 1" chunks. Toss in tapioca starch mixture, then coat in sesame ginger chicken marinade.

5. Heat Fody's Shallot-Infused Olive Oil in a large frying pan or wok until shimmering. Once oil is hot, add in snow peas and cook, about 2 minutes. Then, add cubed chicken thighs and cook over medium-high heat until browned, about 5-7 minutes or until internal temperature reaches 165F.

6. Once the chicken and snow peas are fully cooked, remove from heat and set aside.

7. When rice has finished cooking, remove from heat and add coconut milk, sugar, and a pinch of sea salt, stirring to fully incorporate.

8. Serve with chopped scallion greens as a garnish.

Curried Potato And Parsnip Soup

Ingredients:

- 1 teaspoon gluten-free curry powder, or to taste

- 1 cup (250 ml) low-fat milk, lactose-free milk, or suitable plant-based milk

- Salt and freshly ground black pepper

- Chopped flat-leaf parsley, to garnish

- 1 tablespoon canola oil

- 2 parsnips (14 ounces/400 g), peeled and cut into ¾-inch (2 cm) pieces

- 4 potatoes (1¾ pounds/800 g), peeled and cut into ¾-inch (2 cm) pieces 6½ cups (1.5 liters) gluten-free, onion-free chicken or vegetable stock

Directions:

1. Heat the canola oil in a large heavy-bottomed saucepan over medium heat.

2. Add the parsnips and potatoes and cook, stirring regularly, for 3 to 5 minutes, until lightly golden.

3. Add the stock and bring to a boil. Reduce the heat and simmer for 15 to 20 minutes, stirring occasionally, until the vegetables are tender.

4. Remove from the heat and let cool for about 10 minutes.

5. Puree with an immersion blender (or in batches in a regular blender) until smooth.

6. Add the curry powder and milk and blend again until well combined.

7. Season to taste with salt and pepper.

8. Reheat gently without boiling. Garnish with a sprinkling of parsley and serve.

Carrot And Ginger Soup

Ingredients:

- 6½ cups (1.5 liters) gluten-free, onion-free chicken or vegetable stock

- 1 heaping tablespoon ground ginger

- 1 cup (250 ml) low-fat milk, lactose-free milk, or suitable plant-based milk

- Salt and freshly ground black pepper

- 1 tablespoon olive oil

- 1 small celery root (about 14 ounces/400 g), peeled, halved, and cut into ¼-inch (5 mm) slices

- 4 pounds (1.8 kg) carrots, cut into ¾-inch (2 cm) chunks

- 2 large potatoes (600 g), peeled and cut into quarters

Directions:

1. Heat the olive oil in a large heavy-bottomed saucepan over medium heat, add the celery root, and cook until golden.
2. Add the carrots, potatoes, and stock. Bring to a boil, reduce the heat, cover, and simmer for 20 minutes or until the vegetables are tender.
3. Let cool for about 10 minutes, then puree with an immersion blender (or in batches in a regular blender) until smooth.
4. Stir in the ginger and milk until well combined. You can adjust the quantity of milk depending on how thick you like your soup.
5. Season to taste with salt and pepper. Reheat gently without boiling and serve.

Creamy Seafood Soup

Ingredients:

- ½ cup (125 ml) tomato puree

- ½ fennel bulb, finely chopped

- ½ cup (125 ml) white wine (optional)

- 1 pound (450 g) raw medium shrimp, peeled and deveined

- 2 large or 5 small squid bodies, cleaned and sliced

- 5 ounces (150 g) boneless, skinless firm fish fillets, cut into cubes

- 6 cooked jumbo shrimp

- 1 cup (250 ml) low-fat milk, lactose-free milk, or suitable plant-based milk

- 3 tablespoons (45 g) salted butter

- 2 large carrots, diced

- ½ cup (100 g) long-grain white rice

- 5 cups (1.25 liters) gluten-free, onion-free chicken stock*

- 2 tablespoons plus 2 teaspoons fish sauce, or 4 teaspoons soy sauce plus 2 teaspoons fresh lime juice

- Salt and freshly ground black pepper

- Extra virgin olive oil, to garnish (optional)

Directions:

1. Melt the butter in a large heavy-bottomed saucepan over medium heat. Add the carrots and rice and cook, stirring regularly, for 5 minutes.

2. Add the stock, fish sauce, tomato puree, fennel, and wine (if using) and stir to combine. Bring to a boil, reduce the heat to low, and simmer for 20 minutes, until the rice is tender.

3. Let cool for 10 minutes. Puree with an immersion blender (or in batches in a regular blender) until smooth.

4. Return the pan to the stove over medium heat and bring the soup to a simmer.

5. Add the uncooked shrimp, squid, and fish and simmer for 4 to 5 minutes, until the seafood is just cooked.

6. Add the jumbo shrimp and milk and stir until heated through and combined.

7. Season to taste with salt and pepper, finish with a drizzle of olive oil (if desired), and serve immediately.

Mozzarella Chicken

Ingredients:

- 1 carrot, finely chopped & 400g tin chopped tomatoes

- 3 tbsp tomato purée & 1½ tsp dried oregano

- 85g/3oz pitted green & 2 x 125g packs reduced-fat mozzarella

- 4 chicken breasts, boned and skinned & calorie controlled cooking oil spray

- 1 tbsp garlic infused oil & 1 stalk celery, finely chopped

Directions:

1. Season the bird bosoms with salt and pepper. Splash a large, profound non-stick flameproof skillet or sauté field with oil and notice over high heat.

2. Cook the chook on each facet for 3 mins or until lightly sautéed. Move to a plate.

3. Diminish the warmth to low, splash incredibly more cooking oil into the container and prepare dinner the greens for 4-5mins, mixing until mollified. Include the garlic-mixed oil and cook for more than one moments.

4. Pour inside the tomatoes. Blend within the tomato purée, oregano, and olives. Bring to the bubble and cook dinner for 5mints, mixing continually.

5. Diminish the warm temperature to a sensitive stew and encompass the chook.

6. Cook for 10 minutes, blending now and again till the fowl is delicate and cooked through. Season to flavor.

7. Preheat the flame broil to its most sultry setting.

8. Top the hen and sauce with the cut mozzarella. Sprinkle with ground dark pepper.

9. Set the recent flame broil and cook dinner for 2-3mints or till the cheddar dissolves.

Taco Seasoning

Ingredients:

- 1 ½ teaspoons ground cumin & 1 teaspoon dried oregano

- ½ teaspoon ground black pepper

- 2 tablespoons pure ancho chili powder & 1 tablespoon dried chives

- 2 teaspoons cornstarch or other starch flour & 1 ½ teaspoons salt

Directions:

1. Consolidate all fixings and use as coordinated.

2. To make meat tacos, dark colored 1 lb. ground hamburger and channel oil. Include 2 tablespoons of the flavoring blend and 3/4 cup water.

3. Stew until thickened and bubbly. Ground chicken or turkey might be utilized. For a

more extravagant flavor, take a stab at utilizing my Low-FODMAP Beef Broth rather than water.

4. This flavoring blend formula can be effectively duplicated and put away in a water/air proof holder.

5. Simply measure out 2 tablespoons of the blend per one pound of meat!

Spiced Black Bean & Chicken Soup With Kale

Ingredients:

- 1 tsp chilli flakes

- 400g can chopped tomatoes

- 400g can black beans , rinsed and drained

- 600ml chicken stock

- 175g kale , thick stalks removed, leaves shredded

- 250g leftover roast or ready-cooked chicken

- 50g feta , crumbled, to serve

- 2 tbsp mild olive oil

- 2 fat garlic cloves , crushed

- Small bunch coriander stalks finely chopped, leaves picked

- Zest 1 lime , then cut into wedges

- 2 tsp ground cumin

- Flour & corn tortillas , toasted, to serve

Directions:

1. Heat the oil in a large saucepan, add the garlic, coriander stalks and lime zest, and then fry for 2 mins until fragrant. Stir in the cumin and chilli flakes, fry for 1 min more, and then tip in the tomatoes, beans and stock.

2. Bring to the boil, then crush the beans against the bottom of the pan a few times using a potato masher. This will thicken the soup a little.

3. Stir the kale into the soup, simmer for 5 mins or until tender, then tear in the chicken and let it heat through.

4. Season to taste with salt, pepper and juice from half the lime, then serve in shallow

bowls, scattered with the feta and a few coriander leaves.

5. Serve the remaining lime in wedges for the table, with the toasted tortillas on the side.

6. The longer you leave the chicken in the pan, the thicker the soup will become, so add a splash more stock if you can't serve the soup straight away.

Berry Almond Bakewell

Ingredients:

- 75g self-raising flour, plus a little extra for dusting

- 75g ground almonds

- 150g Total Sweet (xylitol)

- 150g softened butter

- 1 tsp baking powder

- ½ tsp almond extract

- 400g shortcrust pastry cut from a 500g block

- 100g just-thawed frozen raspberries

- 25g flaked almonds

- For the frangipane sponge

- 3 large eggs

Directions:

1. Thinly roll out the pastry on a lightly floured surface , then use it to line the base and sides of a 25cm non-stick, loose-based tart tin.

2. You can leave a little overhang of pastry, but trim away any noticeable excess.

3. Prick the base with a fork and chill for 20 mins. Heat oven to 200C/180C fan/gas 6 and put a baking sheet inside to heat up.

4. Line the pastry case with baking parchment, fill with baking beans and cook on the hot sheet for 10 mins the burst of heat from the baking sheet will help to prevent a soggy bottom.

5. Carefully lift off the paper with the beans and bake for 3 mins more to cook the pastry base.

6. Turn down the oven to 180C/160C fan/gas 4.

7. For the frangipane, put all the ingredients in a large bowl and beat with an electric whisk

until well mixed (alternatively, blitz in a food processor).

8. Scatter the raspberries into the pastry case, spoon over the almond mixture and smooth the top with a knife.

9. Scatter over the flaked almonds and bake for 30-40 mins until golden and firm.

10. Carefully trim any excess pastry from the edge of the tart with a sharp knife before serving.

Kiwi And Oranges Augratin

Ingredients:

- 1 egg yolk

- 1 tablespoon red wine

- 1.5 tablespoons of sugar

- 1 kiwi

- 1 orange

- 0.5 tablespoons of powdered sugar

Directions:

1. Preheat the oven grill.
2. Peel and slice the kiwis and oranges.
3. Arrange the slices on four ovenproof saucers.
4. Heat the egg yolks in a double boiler, adding the wine, a spoonful of cold water, and the sugar.

5. Place the container inside the pot with the hot water.

6. Cook over very low heat, stirring constantly and with a whisk until a thick cream is obtained (about 5 minutes). Spread the cream over the fruit slices in the four saucers.

7. Place the saucers in the oven and cook gratin until a crust forms (about 2-3 minutes).

8. Sprinkle with icing sugar and serve immediately.

Poached Eggs And Ham

Ingredients:

- ½ orange

- 15 g butter

- 2 tablespoons white wine

- 1 tablespoon Cointreau, or Grand Marnier

- (optional)

- 130 g smoked ham, cut into 4 slices

- ½ teaspoon of chives, chopped

- 200g of potatoes

- 3 eggs

- 6 cl of cream cooking

- 5 g dill, chopped

- Salt

- Pepper

- ½ tablespoon olive oil

- ½ tablespoon white vinegar

Directions:

1. Prepare the potato mash
2. Bring to the boil the potatoes whole, without peeling, until very tender (about 20 minutes).
3. Drain them, peel them while still hot, put them in a bowl, and mash them well.
4. In a bowl, beat 2 eggs and then add them to the potatoes. Add the cooking cream, dill, a pinch of salt, and pepper.
5. Mix well and then let it cool until it is compact enough to form two flatbreads.
6. Heat the oil over medium-high heat in a heavy-bottomed skillet. Then put the

flatbreads and cook for 3-4 minutes on the side, until golden brown.

7. Put them on a plate and keep them warm in the oven. Prepare the poached eggs

8. Fill a shallow, large saucepan with water. Add the vinegar and bring to a gentle boil over low heat.

9. Drop one egg at a time into the water. The egg is ready after about 3 minutes when the egg white has completely congealed assuming its white color (the yolk must instead be soft inside). Keep the eggs warm on a plate in the oven Assemble the final dish the flatbreads

10. Place On individual plates (possibly hot), and put a slice of ham on top and the egg on top.

Tomato Soup

Ingredients:

For the Tomato Soup:

- 1/2 tsp white sugar

- 1 tsp red wine vinegar

- 1/4 tsp ground black pepper

- 2 tsps. dried chives

- Salt (to taste)

- 360g tinned chopped tomatoes

- 1 vegetable stock cube dissolved into 1/2 pint of boiling water (suitably low FODMAP)

- 1 tsp dried thyme

- 1 tsp dried oregano

Directions:

1. Preheat your oven to 200C/180C Fan/400F/Gas Mark 6.

2. Place all of your soup Ingredients:into a saucepan and gently simmer for 10-15 mins after which you can either leave it chunky or blend it smooth.

Potato And Leek Soup

Ingredients:

- 1 tsp dried parsley

- 1-2 vegetable stock cubes dissolved in 1 pint of boiling water (suitably low FODMAP)

- Salt and white pepper (to taste)

- 4 tbsps. lactose-free cream (or non-dairy version)

- 2 large potatoes (peeled and diced into small cubes)

- 1 tbsp. butter or vegetable oil

- 100g shredded green leek tips

- ½ tsp dried thyme

Directions:

1. Heat the butter or vegetable oil in a large saucepan, add the leek tips and fry for 2-3 mins.

2. Add the vegetable stock, parsley and potatoes and cook until the potato cubes are soft.

3. Taste the soup, season and add the lactose-free cream before serving.

Campfire Baked Bananas With Caramel Sauce

Ingredients:

- 6 bananas

- 60g coconut shreds

- 60g pecans, chopped

- 120g dark chocolate, broken

For the caramel sauce

- 2 tbsp lactoseor dairy-free butter

- 3 tbsp lactoseor dairy-free cream

- 3 tbsp maple syrup

- 2 tbsp brown sugar

Directions:

1. Slice the bananas down the middle, without cutting through the skin furthest away from you.
2. Stuff the bananas with your fillings of choice pecans, chocolate or coconut and then wrap them individually in foil.
3. Roast them on the barbecue, turning occasionally.
4. Depending how hot your barbecue is, it should take about 1015 minutes for any chocolate to melt and the bananas to soften (check by opening the foil and carefully stabbing with a fork).
5. To make the caramel sauce, melt the maple syrup, sugar, butter and cream together in a small saucepan; set aside.
6. Once the bananas are cooked, transfer to plates, unwrap from the foil and either eat out of the skin or remove the skin and tip onto the plate.

7. Serve with a generous drizzle of caramel sauce.

Salted Peanut Butter Ice Cream

Ingredients:

- 60ml almond milk

- ½ tsp flaky sea salt

- 4 ripe bananas

- 2 tbsp maple syrup

- 3 tbsp peanut butter

Directions:

1. Peel and roughly chop up the bananas. Freeze overnight.
2. In a blender, whizz the bananas up with the maple syrup, peanut butter, almond milk and salt.
3. Serve straight away or spoon into a freezable container for scooping at a later date.

Scrambled Eggs

Ingredients:

- 1/4 teaspoon salt

- Pinch of white pepper

- 4 eggs

- 1/4 cup milk

- 1 tablespoon butter

Directions:

1. Beat the eggs in a bowl.
2. Add the milk and butter, and stir until well combined.
3. Add the salt and white pepper, and mix until well combined.
4. Cook the eggs over medium heat, stirring occasionally, until they are just set and cooked through, about 8 minutes. Serve hot.

Omelet Wraps

Ingredients:

- 1 slice bacon, cooked and crumbled

- 1/4 green onion, sliced

- 1 egg

- 1/4 cup shredded cheddar cheese

Directions:

1. Preheat the oven to 350 degrees F (175 degrees C).
2. Grease a 12x18 inch baking dish.
3. In a medium bowl, whisk together the egg and cheddar cheese.
4. Pour the mixture into the prepared dish.
5. Sprinkle the bacon and green onion over the top of the omelet mixture.

6. Bake for 25 minutes, or until the cheese is melted and bubbly. Serve immediately.

Margherita "Pizzas"

Ingredients:

- ¼ cup coarsely chopped fresh basil

- 2 tablespoons grated Parmesan cheese

- 1 tablespoon olive oil or Garlic-Infused Oil

- 4 Flatbreads for Pizza

- 2 cups tomato sauce

- 4 ounces fresh mozzarella, sliced and drained

Directions:

1. Preheat the oven to 425°F.

2. Place the flatbreads on baking sheets. Top with the tomato sauce, mozzarella, basil, Parmesan, and olive oil.
3. Bake until the cheese is melted and golden, 10 to 12 minutes. Serve immediately.

Deviled Eggs

Ingredients:

- Kosher salt and freshly ground black pepper

- Paprika, for garnish

- Minced fresh chives, for garnish

- ¼ cup mayonnaise

- 1 tablespoon mustard

- Pinch of cayenne pepper

Directions:

1. Put the eggs in a large saucepan. Add enough cold water to cover by 2 inches.
2. Bring to a boil over medium-high heat. Turn off the heat. Cover the pot.
3. Let the eggs sit in the hot water for 15 minutes. Drain the water.
4. When the eggs are cool enough to handle, peel them and cut in half.
5. Separate the yolks from the whites: place the whites on a platter and the yolks in a medium bowl.
6. To the egg yolks, add the mayonnaise, mustard, and cayenne.
7. Mash the egg yolk mixture with a fork until very smooth and light. Season with salt and pepper.
8. Fill the egg whites evenly with the yolk mixture.
9. Sprinkle with paprika and chives for garnish. Serve immediately.

10. The eggs can be cooked in advance. Peel the eggs before storing. Store in a covered container in the refrigerator for up to 3 days.

Basil Omelet With Smashed Tomato

Ingredients:

- 1 tbsp chives, chopped

- ¼ cup shredded mozzarella cheese (or other FODMAP-approved cheese)

- 1-2 basil leaves, chopped finely

- 2 tomatoes, halved

- 3 eggs

- Pepper

Directions:

1. Break the eggs into a bowl and add a splash of water.
2. Whisk the mixture with a fork and add the chives and a pinch of pepper. Set aside.
3. Place the halved tomatoes on til in a hot skillet on the stove or onto a hot grill on low

to medium heat. Turn occasionally until they are starting to char, then remove them and place them on plates. Squish slightly so that the juices are released.

4. Take the egg mixture and whisk it slightly before pouring it into a hot pan on medium heat.

5. Leave the mixture for a few seconds before gently stirring the uncooked egg until it is cooked but still slightly loose.

6. Place the cheese and a basil leaf on one half of the egg and then gently fold the omelet in half.

7. Let it cook for another minute. Once it is cooked, cut the omelet in half and serve with the tomato.

Eggs In Clouds

Ingredients:

- ¼ cup chives, chopped

- ¼ cup parmesan cheese, shredded

- 4 eggs

Directions:

1. Separate egg whites from the yolks. Whisk egg whites for 5 minutes.
2. Add chives and cheese. Mix well.
3. Divide egg white mixture into 4 and arrange them in a baking tray lined with parchment paper. Bake for 3 minutes.
4. Place the yolks on in the center of each egg white. Cook for another 2 minutes.

Scrambled Eggs

Ingredients:

- 2 eggs

- 30 g butter

- Salt and ground black pepper

Directions:

1. Beat the eggs with salt including pepper using a fork.

2. Melt the butter in a nonstick skillet over medium heat. Look closely: butter does not turn golden!

3. Pour the eggs to the pan and mix for 1-2 minutes until they are creamy and cooked a little less than you like.

4. Get that the eggs will continue to cook even once you put them on your plate.

5. Tips!

6. These creamy eggs, pair well with many popular low carb dishes.

7. Of course, there is the option of eating them with classic accompaniments such as bacon or sausage, but there are other great options such as salmon, avocado, cold cuts and cheese (cheddar, fresh mozzarella or feta).

8. And if you're very hungry (or are cooking with large eggs), do not be shy: use more butter!

Fody's Cheesy Gordita Crunch Copycat

Ingredients:

- FODMAP tortillas if following the diet)

- 4-6 hard shell corn taco shells

- 1 cup shredded cheddar cheese

- Shredded lettuce

- Fody's Mild Salsa

- ¼ cup

- Fody's Garden Herb Dressing

- 2 tbsp sour cream or greek yogurt

- 1 lb ground beef

- 1 tbsp olive oil

- 1 tbsp Fody's Taco Seasoning

- ⅓ cup

- Fody's Taco Sauce

- 4-6 small soft corn tortillas (opt for Low

Directions:

1. Pre-heat oven to 375F.
2. In a large skillet over medium high heat, drizzle Fody Olive Oil + heat till simmering. Add in ground beef and Fody Taco Seasoning, breaking up ground beef with a spatula.
3. Allow ground beef to brown approximately 7 minutes, then add Fody Taco Sauce, continuing to break up beef as it browns.
4. While beef finishes, grease a lined baking sheet and arrange soft corn tortillas on it.
5. Sprinkle shredded cheddar cheese evenly onto each tortilla, then sprinkle additional Fody Taco seasoning on top of cheese. (Remember to stick with 2 oz or less of a low

lactose cheese, if following the Low FODMAP diet).

6. Bake for 3-4 minutes until the cheese is beginning to melt. Remove tray from oven + add hard taco shells by placing one side down onto the melted cheese. Bake an additional 2 minutes, then press the cheese side on to the hard shell tortilla and bake an additional 2 minutes to set.

7. Before assembling tacos, in a small mixing bowl, mix up Fody Garden Herb dressing and sour cream/greek yogurt for your cheesy gordita crunch sauce recipe.

8. Once shells are set, divide ground beef up into each taco shell + top with shredded lettuce, Fody Mild Salsa and sour cream Garden Herb dressing.

Quiche Lorraine

Ingredients:

For the crust

- ½ cup/ 70 gr. rice flour & ½ cup/ 70 gr. millet flour

- ½ cup/ 75 gr. tapioca starch & ½ tsp salt

- 4 tbsp butter & 1 tbsp apple cider vinegar

- 4 to 6 tbsp water

For the filling

- 3,5 oz/ 100gr bacon, finely chopped

- 2 eggs & 2 tbsp greek yogurt

- ½ cup/140ml lactose-free milk

- 1,4 oz/ 40 gr. swiss cheese (gruyère), diced or grated

- ½ tsp nutmeg & A little pinch of salt

- Black pepper to taste

Directions:

1. For the outside, place flours, starch, margarine, and salt in a bowl.

2. Utilizing your fingers, rub fixings together until pea-size disintegrates structure. Include the vinegar and one tablespoon of water at once and manipulate until mixture structures.

3. Consistency ought to be flexible and smooth, so include more water if necessary.

4. Structure the mixture into a ball and chill until you've finished stages 2 and 3.

5. Add the hacked bacon to a non-stick container and sauté over medium warmth for 5 minutes or until firm.

6. Put aside to cool.

7. In a bowl whisk the eggs, greek yogurt, and milk. Include the cheddar, nutmeg, salt, pepper lastly the cooled bacon.

8. In one major or 4 little tart skillet, move the batter to the focal point of the container and press with your fingers out to the edges of the dish, at that point up the sides until it takes after an outside layer.

9. Squeeze an alluring lip around the edge of the dish and prick the base of the hull done with a fork. Fill in with the fluid blend.

10. Preheat stove to 350ºF/180ºC and heat for 50 minutes.

11. Enable the quiche to cool for a couple of minutes before serving.

12. Appreciate hot or cold with a green serving of mixed greens and... bon appétit!

Sardine Spaghetti With Tomato-Caper Sauce

Ingredients:

- Salt and freshly ground black pepper & 3 oz (about 3 big handfuls) spinach leaves

- 2 to 3 scallions, sliced & ¼ tsp red chile flakes

- 1 (14.5 oz) can petite diced tomatoes & 1 tbsp drained capers, roughly chopped

- 6 oz gluten-free spaghetti & ¼ to ½ avocado, chopped

- 2 (4.37 oz) cans sardines, drained and de-boned if necessary

- 2 tbsp extra-virgin olive oil & 3 tbsp gluten-free breadcrumbs

- Lemon wedges for serving

Directions:

1. Boil 2 tbsp of the oil in a big skillet on medium.

2. Add breadcrumbs and mix to coat with oil. Cook, mixing by the way till daintily toasted, round 3 minutes. Season with salt and pepper to flavor. Move to a touch bowl and put in a secure spot.

3. In a similar skillet, warmness 1 tbsp of the oil on medium warmth. Include spinach and season with dark pepper to taste.

4. Cook, mixing every on occasion until contracted, around 2 minutes. Move to every other bowl and put in a safe spot.

5. Add staying 1 tbsp oil to a comparable skillet and warmth on medium. Include scallions and stew drops and prepare dinner till scallion is sensitive around 1 second.

6. Include tomatoes with their juice. Raise warmth to medium-excessive and produce to

a stew. Cook, mixing every so often, till sauce thickens marginally, 8 to ten mins. Mix in escapades and expel from warm temperature.

7. Then, warmness a large pot of water to the point of boiling on excessive warmness. Season with salt and consist of spaghetti.

8. Cook till still incredibly firm as per package deal headings and channel.

9. Return pasta to the pot you certainly cooked it in. Include sardines, spinach and tomato sauce (for low-FODMAP, hold approximately ¼ cup of the sauce for some other users).

10. Spot the pot over low warmth and blend delicately to enroll in. Cook just until warmed through, 1 to two minutes. Top every offering with breadcrumbs and avocado and present with lemon wedges.

www.ingramcontent.com/pod-product-compliance
Lightning Source LLC
Chambersburg PA
CBHW060233030426
42335CB00014B/1429